Low Oxalate Diet for Beginners

Understanding the Importance of Low Oxalate Diet

By

Alasdair Ciaran

Table of Contents

CHAPTER 1

Introduction

1.1 What Are Oxalates?

Oxalates, also known as oxalic acid, are naturally occurring compounds found in a wide variety of plant-based foods. Chemically, oxalates are organic acids that belong to a group of molecules called oxalate salts. These compounds are composed of carbon, hydrogen, and oxygen atoms, with two carbon atoms linked together ($C_2H_2O_4$). Oxalates can be either soluble or insoluble in water, depending on their chemical form and the specific minerals they combine with.

In the context of human nutrition, oxalates are noteworthy because they have the ability to form insoluble crystals when they combine with certain minerals, primarily calcium, in the body. These crystals are known as calcium oxalate crystals. The formation of these crystals can occur both in the urinary tract (kidneys and bladder) and elsewhere in the body, and this process plays a central role in the discussion of why oxalates matter.

1.2 Why Do Oxalates Matter?

Understanding the significance of oxalates involves recognizing their dual role in human health, as both dietary components and potential health concerns:

A. Dietary Components:

Oxalates are present in a wide range of foods that are commonly consumed as part of a healthy diet. These foods include leafy greens (such as spinach and kale), nuts and seeds, some fruits (like rhubarb and blackberries), chocolate, and certain grains. Many of these foods are rich in essential nutrients and offer various health benefits, so it's important to strike a balance when considering their inclusion in your diet.

B. Health Concerns:

The concern with oxalates arises primarily due to their potential to contribute to the formation of calcium oxalate crystals, which can lead to various health issues, including:

1. **Kidney Stones:** When calcium oxalate crystals accumulate in

the kidneys, they can combine and form solid masses known as kidney stones. These stones can be extremely painful and may require medical intervention for removal.

2. **Hyperoxaluria:** Some individuals have a condition called hyperoxaluria, where they produce an excessive amount of oxalates or have difficulty metabolizing them effectively. This condition can increase the risk of kidney stone formation.

3. **Digestive Issues:** In rare cases, high oxalate intake can lead to digestive issues, such as irritation of the gastrointestinal tract, as oxalates can bind to minerals in the digestive system

and potentially interfere with nutrient absorption.

4. **Nutrient Interactions:** Oxalates can bind with minerals, particularly calcium, in the digestive tract, potentially reducing the absorption of these essential nutrients. This can affect calcium availability for bone health, among other concerns.

while oxalates can pose health risks for some individuals, they are not inherently harmful to everyone. Many people can consume oxalate-containing foods without any issues. The key to managing oxalates is understanding your individual health profile, consulting with a healthcare professional if needed, and making informed dietary choices based on your specific needs and risk factors.

oxalates are natural compounds found in a variety of foods, and their significance lies in their potential to form calcium oxalate crystals, which can lead to kidney stones and other health concerns for some individuals. Balancing oxalate intake and considering individual health factors are crucial when addressing the role of oxalates in your diet.

CHAPTER 2

Getting Started with a Low Oxalate Diet

2.1 Assessing Your Current Diet

Before embarking on a low oxalate diet, it's essential to assess your current eating habits and understand your dietary patterns. This step will help you identify high oxalate foods that you may need to reduce or eliminate. Here's how to go about it:

- **Food Journal:** Keep a detailed food journal for at least a week, documenting everything you eat and drink. Include portion sizes and meal times.

- **Oxalate Content:** Use reliable resources or apps that provide oxalate content information for various foods. This will help you identify which items in your diet are high in oxalates.

- **Symptoms:** Take note of any symptoms you may have experienced, such as kidney stones or digestive discomfort, as these could be related to your oxalate intake.

2.2 Setting Your Goals

Once you have a clear understanding of your current diet, you can set specific goals for transitioning to a low oxalate eating plan. Your goals should be realistic and tailored to your individual needs and circumstances:

- **Reduction Targets:** Determine how much you want to reduce your oxalate intake. Some people opt for a moderate reduction, while others may need to follow a very low oxalate diet, especially if they have a history of kidney stones or hyperoxaluria.

- **Health Objectives:** Define the health objectives you want to achieve through a low oxalate diet. This could include preventing kidney stones, managing specific medical conditions, or reducing digestive discomfort.

- **Timeframe:** Decide on a timeframe for achieving your goals. Depending on your objectives, you may opt for gradual changes or a more rapid transition.

2.3 Creating a Plan

With your goals in mind, it's time to develop a practical and sustainable plan for transitioning to a low oxalate diet:

- **Educate Yourself:** Learn about the oxalate content of common foods. Reliable resources, dietary guidelines, and books on low oxalate diets can provide valuable information.

- **Food Lists:** Compile lists of high, moderate, and low oxalate foods. These lists will serve as references when planning your meals.

- **Meal Planning:** Design a meal plan that incorporates low oxalate foods while minimizing or eliminating high oxalate choices. Ensure that your meals are balanced and provide essential nutrients.

- **Grocery Shopping:** Make a shopping list based on your meal plan. Prioritize low oxalate foods and familiarize yourself with alternatives to high oxalate ingredients.

- **Food Preparation:** Explore low oxalate cooking techniques and recipes to make your meals enjoyable. Experiment with herbs and spices to enhance flavor.

- **Hydration:** Consider your fluid intake, as adequate

hydration is important for kidney health. Water is typically the best choice, but consult your healthcare provider for personalized recommendations.

- **Support System:** If necessary, inform your family or housemates about your dietary changes and enlist their support in maintaining a low oxalate environment.

- **Consult a Healthcare Professional:** If you have specific medical conditions or dietary concerns, it's advisable to consult a registered dietitian or healthcare provider. They can offer personalized guidance and monitor your progress.

Transitioning to a low oxalate diet is a process, and it may take time to adjust to new eating habits. Be patient with yourself, monitor your progress, and make adjustments as needed to ensure that your diet remains balanced and nutritionally adequate.

2.4 Stocking Your Kitchen

One of the keys to success on a low oxalate diet is having the right foods readily available in your kitchen. Here's how to stock your kitchen for a low oxalate diet:

- **Low Oxalate Staples:** Purchase low oxalate staples such as low oxalate grains (e.g., rice, quinoa), lean proteins (e.g., chicken, fish), low oxalate vegetables (e.g., cauliflower, broccoli), and low oxalate fruits (e.g., apples, pears).

- **Dairy and Alternatives:** If you tolerate dairy, stock up on low oxalate dairy products like milk and yogurt. If you're lactose intolerant or prefer dairy alternatives, choose low oxalate options like almond milk or lactose-free yogurt.

- **Fresh Herbs and Spices:** Use fresh herbs and spices to flavor your meals. These can add variety and enhance the taste of low oxalate dishes.

- **Nuts and Seeds:** If you're not entirely eliminating nuts and seeds, opt for lower oxalate options such as pine nuts, sunflower seeds, or flaxseeds.

- **Cooking Oils:** Keep cooking oils like olive oil, canola oil, or avocado oil on hand for sautéing and salad dressings.

- **Low Oxalate Snacks:** Have low oxalate snacks available for when you need a quick bite. Options may include rice cakes, rice crackers, or carrot sticks with hummus.

- **Herbal Teas:** If you enjoy tea, consider stocking up on herbal teas like chamomile, peppermint, or ginger, which are generally low in oxalates.

- **Oxalate-Free Water:** Ensure you have access to oxalate-free water for drinking. Some tap water sources may contain oxalates, so using a water filter can be helpful.

- **Storage Containers:** Invest in good quality storage containers to help keep your low oxalate ingredients fresh and organized.

2.5 Meal Planning and Preparation Tips

Effective meal planning and preparation are essential for maintaining a low oxalate diet and making it a sustainable part of your lifestyle. Here are some tips to help you succeed:

- **Plan Ahead:** Plan your meals for the week, taking into account your low oxalate goals and dietary preferences.

- **Batch Cooking:** Prepare larger quantities of low oxalate dishes and freeze them in individual portions. This makes it easier to have low oxalate meals on hand when you're short on time.

- **Experiment with Recipes:** Explore low oxalate recipes online or in cookbooks to keep your meals interesting and flavorful.

- **Variety is Key:** Don't stick to the same foods day in and day out. Incorporate a wide variety of low oxalate foods to ensure you get a range of nutrients.

- **Label Reading:** When shopping for packaged foods, carefully read food labels to check for oxalate content. Look for products labeled as "low oxalate."

- **Portion Control:** Be mindful of portion sizes. Even low oxalate foods can contribute to oxalate intake if consumed in excess.

- **Stay Hydrated:** Drink plenty of water throughout the day to help flush out any excess oxalates in your system.

- **Prep Snacks:** Have low oxalate snacks, such as sliced fruits or veggies, prepped and ready to grab when hunger strikes.

- **Dine Out with Care:** When dining at restaurants, inquire about menu options and preparation methods. Request modifications if needed to make dishes low oxalate.

- **Track Your Progress:** Consider keeping a food diary to track your low oxalate meals,

symptoms, and any changes in
your health.

- **Seek Support:** Join online
  forums or support groups for
  individuals following low
  oxalate diets. Sharing
  experiences and tips with others
  can be motivating and
  informative.

Transitioning to a low oxalate diet is a
journey that requires patience and
flexibility. Over time, you'll become
more familiar with low oxalate foods
and find strategies that work best for
you in meal planning and preparation.
Consulting with a healthcare provider
or dietitian can also provide valuable
guidance tailored to your specific
needs and goals.

CHAPTER 3

Foods High and Low in Oxalates

3.1 High-Oxalate Foods to Avoid

Leafy Greens

Leafy greens are often considered a staple of a healthy diet due to their rich nutrient content. However, many leafy greens are also high in oxalates, which may be a concern for individuals with certain health conditions. Here are some high-oxalate leafy greens to be cautious of:

- **Spinach:** Spinach is notorious for its high oxalate content. While it's a good source of various vitamins and minerals, it's advisable to consume it in moderation on a low oxalate diet.

- **Kale:** Kale, another popular leafy green, contains significant amounts of oxalates. If you enjoy kale, consider using it sparingly or opting for lower oxalate greens.

- **Collard Greens:** Collard greens are also relatively high in oxalates. If you're a fan of collard greens, be mindful of portion sizes.

Nuts and Seeds

Nuts and seeds are nutrient-dense snacks, but many varieties are high in oxalates. Here are some examples of high-oxalate nuts and seeds:

- **Almonds:** Almonds are a popular nut but contain a substantial amount of oxalates. Consider alternative nuts like cashews or macadamia nuts that are lower in oxalates.

- **Peanuts:** While technically legumes, peanuts are often grouped with nuts and have a moderate oxalate content. If you consume peanut products like peanut butter, do so in moderation.

- **Sesame Seeds:** Sesame seeds and tahini (sesame paste) have high oxalate levels. Explore other seed options such as flaxseeds or chia seeds, which are lower in oxalates.

Whole Grains

Whole grains are generally recommended for their fiber and nutrient content, but some grains contain notable levels of oxalates:

- **Whole Wheat:** Whole wheat products, including whole wheat bread and pasta, have a moderate oxalate content. If you're following a strict low oxalate diet, you may need to limit your intake of these foods.

- **Bran:** Bran from grains like wheat, rice, and oats is high in oxalates. Consider refined grains or grain alternatives if you're looking to reduce oxalate intake.

Fruits

While fruits are an essential part of a balanced diet, some fruits contain significant oxalate levels:

- **Rhubarb:** Rhubarb is exceptionally high in oxalates and should be avoided or consumed sparingly if you're following a low oxalate diet.

- **Blackberries:** Blackberries have a moderate oxalate content. If you enjoy berries, consider opting for lower oxalate options like blueberries or strawberries.

Chocolate and Cocoa

Chocolate and cocoa products, beloved by many, are rich in oxalates:

- **Dark Chocolate:** Dark chocolate, in particular,

contains high levels of oxalates.
If you have a sweet tooth,
consider indulging in lower
oxalate treats occasionally.

3.2 Low-Oxalate Foods to Include

Proteins

Protein sources that are typically low in oxalates include:

- **Lean Meats:** Lean cuts of beef, pork, poultry, and fish are excellent sources of protein without significant oxalate content.

- **Eggs:** Eggs are naturally low in oxalates and can be included in various dishes.

- **Tofu:** Tofu and other soy-based products are generally low in oxalates and suitable for vegetarians and vegans.

Vegetables

Many vegetables are low in oxalates and can be freely included in a low oxalate diet:

- **Cauliflower:** Cauliflower is a versatile low oxalate vegetable that can be used in place of high oxalate alternatives like spinach.

- **Broccoli:** Broccoli is another low oxalate cruciferous vegetable that offers a range of nutrients.

- **Carrots:** Carrots are a nutritious root vegetable with minimal oxalate content.

Fruits

Several fruits have low oxalate levels and can be enjoyed as part of a low oxalate diet:

- **Apples:** Apples are low in oxalates and provide dietary fiber and vitamins.

- **Pears:** Pears are another low oxalate fruit option that adds variety to your diet.

Dairy and Dairy Alternatives

Dairy products and alternatives that are typically low in oxalates include:

- **Milk:** Regular cow's milk is a good source of calcium and protein and is generally low in oxalates.

- **Lactose-Free Options:** If you're lactose intolerant,

lactose-free milk and dairy products are low in oxalates and can be included.

Grains and Starches

Select grains and starches that are naturally low in oxalates:

- **White Rice:** White rice is a low oxalate grain and can be used as a base for various dishes.

- **Potatoes:** Potatoes are a low oxalate starchy vegetable that can be enjoyed in various preparations.

understanding the oxalate content of different food groups is crucial for effectively managing a low oxalate diet. By being aware of high-oxalate foods to avoid and low-oxalate foods to include, individuals can make informed dietary choices that align with their specific health needs and goals. Remember to consult with a healthcare professional or dietitian for personalized guidance and to ensure your diet remains balanced and nutritionally adequate.

CHAPTER 4

Planning Balanced Low Oxalate Meals

Planning balanced low oxalate meals is essential to ensure you meet your nutritional needs while managing your oxalate intake. Building a balanced plate involves considering various food groups and portion sizes. Here's how to create balanced low oxalate meals:

4.1 Building a Balanced Plate

When constructing a balanced low oxalate plate, aim to include a variety of food groups to provide essential nutrients. Here's a breakdown of what your plate should ideally look like:

1. Low Oxalate Vegetables (Fill Half Your Plate): Fill half of your plate with a variety of low oxalate vegetables. These should be the foundation of your meal. Examples of low oxalate vegetables include cauliflower, broccoli, carrots, zucchini, and bell peppers.

2. Protein (One-Quarter of Your Plate): Dedicate one-quarter of your plate to a source of protein. Choose lean meats, poultry, fish, tofu, or legumes (e.g., lentils, chickpeas) to meet your protein needs. These options are generally low in oxalates.

3. Low Oxalate Grains or Starches (One-Quarter of Your Plate): The other quarter of your plate can be filled with low oxalate grains or starches. Options include white rice, potatoes, or low oxalate pasta. These foods provide energy and can help you feel satisfied.

4. Healthy Fats (Incorporate Sparingly): Incorporate healthy fats in small quantities. You can use a drizzle of olive oil on your vegetables, add some avocado slices, or sprinkle nuts like cashews (if tolerated) for flavor and healthy fats.

5. Dairy or Dairy Alternatives (If Tolerated): If you tolerate dairy, consider adding a small serving of low oxalate dairy or dairy alternatives to your meal. This can provide calcium and other nutrients. Examples include a glass of lactose-free milk or a serving of plain Greek yogurt.

6. Seasonings and Flavor Enhancers: Use herbs, spices, and seasonings to enhance the flavor of your meal without relying on high oxalate ingredients. Fresh herbs like basil or thyme and spices like paprika or cumin can add depth to your dishes.

7. Hydration: Remember to hydrate yourself with water throughout your meal. Adequate hydration is essential for kidney health and can help dilute any oxalates in your system.

8. Portion Control: Pay attention to portion sizes. While low oxalate foods are generally safe, consuming large quantities of any food group can lead to an imbalance in your diet.

Sample Balanced Low Oxalate Meals:

- Grilled chicken breast with steamed broccoli and white rice.

- Baked salmon with a side of roasted carrots and mashed potatoes (with skin removed).

- Lentil and vegetable stir-fry with tofu served over white rice.

- A salad with mixed greens, cherry tomatoes, cucumber, and a small portion of low oxalate cheese (if tolerated). Dress with olive oil and lemon juice.

- Scrambled eggs with sautéed spinach (in moderation) and a slice of toast made from low oxalate bread.

Individual dietary needs can vary, and it's important to tailor your meals to your specific health goals and tolerances. If you have specific medical conditions or dietary restrictions, consult with a healthcare provider or dietitian to create a personalized and balanced low oxalate meal plan that meets your unique needs.

Breakfast Ideas:

Option 1: Low Oxalate Oatmeal

- Cooked rolled oats (low oxalate) topped with fresh sliced strawberries (in moderation) and a drizzle of honey or maple syrup.

- A side of scrambled eggs.

Option 2: Greek Yogurt Parfait

- Plain Greek yogurt (if tolerated) layered with blueberries and chopped almonds (in moderation).

- Sprinkle with cinnamon for added flavor.

Option 3: Breakfast Burrito

- Scrambled eggs with diced bell peppers, onions, and tomatoes (low oxalate).

- Wrap the mixture in a low oxalate tortilla or serve as a bowl.

Lunch Suggestions:

Option 1: Grilled Chicken Salad

- Grilled chicken breast over a bed of mixed greens, cherry tomatoes, and cucumber.

- Dress with olive oil and balsamic vinegar.

Option 2: Lentil Soup

- Homemade or store-bought low oxalate lentil soup.

- Serve with a side of low oxalate crackers.

Option 3: Quinoa Bowl

- Quinoa (low oxalate) with roasted vegetables (e.g., cauliflower, broccoli, carrots).

- Top with a tahini dressing (low oxalate).

Dinner Recipes:

Option 1: Baked Salmon with Asparagus

- Baked salmon fillet seasoned with lemon, dill, and black pepper.

- Served with roasted asparagus (low oxalate) and a side of white rice.

Option 2: Chicken Stir-Fry

- Sautéed chicken breast with low oxalate vegetables like bell peppers, snow peas, and carrots.

- Serve over white rice or rice noodles (low oxalate).

Option 3: Turkey and Vegetable Skewers

- Skewer pieces of turkey breast, zucchini, and cherry tomatoes.

- Grill or bake and serve with a quinoa salad (low oxalate) with herbs and lemon vinaigrette.

Snack Options:

Option 1: Cottage Cheese with Pineapple

- Low oxalate cottage cheese topped with fresh pineapple chunks (in moderation).

Option 2: Veggie Sticks with Hummus

- Sliced cucumbers, carrots, and bell peppers served with a side of low oxalate hummus.

Option 3: Rice Cakes with Almond Butter

- Low oxalate rice cakes spread with almond butter (if tolerated) and a drizzle of honey.

Adjust portion sizes and ingredients based on your specific dietary needs and preferences. Additionally, be mindful of portion control to maintain a balanced low oxalate diet. If you have medical conditions that require strict oxalate restrictions, consult with a healthcare provider or dietitian for personalized meal plans and guidance.

4.2 Low Oxalate Vegetables

Low oxalate vegetables are a crucial component of a low oxalate diet. These vegetables are typically safe for individuals who need to limit oxalate intake due to kidney stones or related conditions. Some examples of low oxalate vegetables include:

- **Bell Peppers:** Bell peppers, whether red, green, or yellow, are low in oxalates and can be used in various dishes.

- **Cauliflower:** Cauliflower is a versatile low oxalate vegetable that can be used to make a variety of dishes, from cauliflower rice to roasted cauliflower.

- **Zucchini:** Zucchini is another low oxalate vegetable that can be used in spiralized form for pasta alternatives or simply sautéed.

- **Cabbage:** Cabbage, whether in coleslaw or stir-fry, is a low oxalate option.

- **Carrots:** Carrots are low in oxalates and can be consumed in various ways, including raw or as part of stews and soups.

- **Onions:** Onions are low oxalate vegetables that add flavor to many dishes without contributing to oxalate intake.

- **Green Beans:** Green beans are a popular side dish and are low in oxalates.

Cooking methods can affect the oxalate content of vegetables. Boiling and draining vegetables can reduce their oxalate levels, making them even more suitable for a low oxalate diet.

4.3 Low Oxalate Grains

Grains are a significant part of many diets, and it's important for those following a low oxalate diet to choose grains that are low in oxalates. Here are some examples of low oxalate grains:

- **White Rice:** White rice is a low oxalate alternative to brown rice, which contains higher levels of oxalates.

- **Quinoa:** Quinoa is a relatively low oxalate grain and is often considered a healthy substitute for rice or other grains.

- **Oats:** Rolled oats and steel-cut oats are generally low in oxalates, making them a suitable option for breakfast or baking.

- **Barley:** Pearl barley and hulled barley are low oxalate grains that can be used in soups and stews.

- **Amaranth:** Amaranth is a pseudograin that is low in oxalates and can be used as a side dish or in recipes.

- **Millet:** Millet is another low oxalate grain that can be used as a base for various dishes.

It's important to note that while these grains are generally low in oxalates, oxalate content can vary, so it's advisable to consume them in moderation and monitor individual tolerance.

4.4 Low Oxalate Proteins

Protein sources play a vital role in a balanced diet, and it's possible to incorporate low oxalate protein options into a low oxalate diet. Here are some examples:

- **Chicken:** Skinless chicken breast is a low oxalate protein source and can be prepared in numerous ways.

- **Turkey:** Turkey is another lean protein option that is generally low in oxalates.

- **Fish:** Many types of fish, such as salmon, cod, and haddock, are low in oxalates and provide healthy omega-3 fatty acids.

- **Eggs:** Eggs are a versatile and low oxalate protein source, suitable for breakfast or as an ingredient in various dishes.

- **Tofu:** Tofu is a plant-based protein option that is low in oxalates and can be used in both savory and sweet dishes.

- **Lean Beef:** Lean cuts of beef, like sirloin or tenderloin, contain fewer oxalates compared to fatty cuts.

When choosing protein sources, it's essential to select lean cuts and practice healthy cooking methods like grilling, baking, or poaching to minimize added fats, which can contribute to kidney stone formation.

4.5 Low Oxalate Dairy

Dairy products can be part of a low oxalate diet, as long as you choose low oxalate options. Here are some examples of low oxalate dairy products:

- **Milk:** Most cow's milk is considered low in oxalates,

making it a suitable choice for those who enjoy dairy.

- **Yogurt:** Plain, unflavored yogurt is generally low in oxalates and can be a nutritious addition to your diet.

- **Cheese:** Some types of cheese, such as cheddar and mozzarella, are relatively low in oxalates and can be enjoyed in moderation.

- **Butter:** Butter, used in moderation, is a low oxalate fat source that can be used for cooking and baking.

It's worth noting that not all dairy products are low in oxalates. Some dairy alternatives like almond milk or soy-based products may be higher in oxalates, so it's important to read labels and choose wisely.

4.6 Low Oxalate Beverages

Beverages can also contribute to your oxalate intake, so it's important to choose low oxalate options when following a low oxalate diet. Here are some examples:

- **Water:** Water is the best choice for maintaining hydration and minimizing oxalate intake.

- **Herbal Teas:** Many herbal teas, such as chamomile or peppermint, are low in oxalates and can be enjoyed as caffeine-free alternatives.

- **Fruit Juices:** Some fruit juices, like apple and pear juice, are lower in oxalates compared to citrus juices, but they should still be consumed in moderation.

- **Milk:** As mentioned earlier, most cow's milk is considered low in oxalates, making it a suitable beverage choice.

- **Coffee and Tea:** Coffee and tea are generally low in oxalates, but it's important to consider any added ingredients, like cream or sugar, which may affect the oxalate content.

While these beverages are generally low in oxalates, individual tolerances can vary, so it's a good practice to monitor your response to different beverages and make adjustments as needed.

when following a low oxalate diet, it's crucial to maintain a balanced and varied diet to ensure you're getting the necessary nutrients for overall health. Consult with a healthcare professional or dietitian for personalized guidance and to address any specific dietary concerns.

CHAPTER 5

Cooking and Dining Out

5.1 Cooking Techniques to Reduce Oxalates

Cooking can alter the oxalate content of certain foods. Here are some techniques to help reduce oxalates in your meals:

- **Boiling:** Boiling vegetables can leach out some of their oxalate content into the cooking water. Discard the water to reduce oxalate levels. This works well for vegetables like spinach and kale.

- **Blanching:** Similar to boiling, blanching involves briefly immersing vegetables in boiling water, followed by rapid cooling in ice water. This method can help reduce oxalates while retaining color and texture.

- **Steaming:** Steaming vegetables can be an effective way to retain their nutrients while reducing oxalates. Just be sure not to overcook them.

- **Peeling and Discarding:** In some cases, peeling and discarding the outer layers of certain vegetables can help reduce oxalate content. For instance, peeling potatoes before boiling them can lower oxalate levels.

- **Soaking and Draining:**
  Soaking grains, legumes, or
  seeds overnight and then
  draining them can reduce their
  oxalate content. Rinse them
  thoroughly before cooking.

5.2 Low Oxalate Cooking Tips

Here are some additional cooking tips
to help you maintain a low oxalate
diet:

- **Use Low Oxalate Substitutes:**
  Replace high oxalate
  ingredients with low oxalate
  alternatives. For instance, opt
  for cauliflower rice instead of
  traditional rice or mashed
  potatoes instead of mashed
  sweet potatoes.

- **Limit High Oxalate Spices:** Some spices, like cinnamon and turmeric, are high in oxalates. Use them sparingly or consider alternative seasonings.

- **Homemade Sauces and Dressings:** When making sauces and dressings, prepare them at home using low oxalate ingredients. This gives you more control over the oxalate content.

- **Dilution:** Dilute high oxalate foods with low oxalate counterparts. For example, mix high oxalate spinach with low oxalate lettuce in salads.

- **Consider Oxalate Binders:** Consult with a healthcare provider about oxalate binder medications if you have a medical condition that requires strict oxalate control.

5.3 Navigating Restaurants and Fast Food

Eating out while following a low oxalate diet can be a bit challenging, but it's manageable with some careful choices:

- **Review Menus Online:** Before going to a restaurant, check their menu online if available. Look for dishes that are likely to be low in oxalates, such as grilled meats or salads with low oxalate vegetables.

- **Ask Questions:** When dining out, don't hesitate to ask your server about ingredient options and preparation methods. Request modifications to suit your dietary needs, such as substituting high oxalate sides with low oxalate options.

- **Choose Simple Preparations:** Select dishes that have simple preparations with fewer ingredients, as they are less likely to contain high oxalate components.

- **Beware of Sauces and Dressings:** Be cautious about sauces, dressings, and condiments as they may contain hidden high oxalate ingredients. Ask for them on the side so you can control the quantity.

- **Fast Food Considerations:** When opting for fast food,

choose items that are less likely
to be high in oxalates, such as
grilled chicken sandwiches
without spinach or salads
without high oxalate toppings.

- **BYO (Bring Your Own):** If
you're concerned about finding
low oxalate options, consider
bringing your own low oxalate
snacks or side dishes to
supplement your meal.

- **Stay Informed:** Stay informed
about popular chain restaurants
that offer allergen or nutrition
guides. These guides can help
you identify low oxalate
choices.

Communication with restaurant staff
is essential to ensure your dietary
needs are met. If you're unsure about
menu items, it's always best to ask

questions and request modifications to accommodate your low oxalate diet.

CHAPTER 6
Managing Special Dietary Needs

Managing special dietary needs on a low oxalate diet can be challenging, especially for vegetarians and vegans or picky eaters. Here are some tips for addressing these specific situations:

6.1 Low Oxalate Diet for Vegetarians and Vegans

Following a low oxalate diet as a vegetarian or vegan requires careful planning to ensure you meet your nutritional needs. Here are some strategies to help:

- **Diversify Protein Sources:**
  Incorporate a variety of low
  oxalate plant-based proteins
  such as tofu, tempeh, legumes
  (e.g., lentils, chickpeas), and
  edamame. These options
  provide essential nutrients
  while being lower in oxalates
  compared to high oxalate
  animal proteins.

- **opt for Low Oxalate
  Vegetables:** Focus on low
  oxalate vegetables like
  cauliflower, broccoli, zucchini,
  and bell peppers. These can
  serve as the foundation of your
  meals.

- **Use Low Oxalate Grains:**
  Choose low oxalate grains like
  white rice, quinoa, and
  couscous as your primary

carbohydrate sources. Be mindful of portion sizes.

- **Plan Balanced Meals:** Ensure your meals are well-balanced by combining low oxalate ingredients from various food groups. For example, a tofu stir-fry with broccoli, bell peppers, and white rice can be a nutritious option.

- **Homemade Veggie Burgers:** Make homemade veggie burgers using low oxalate ingredients like chickpeas, lentils, or black beans. This way, you can control the oxalate content.

- **Explore Low Oxalate Dairy Alternatives:** If you tolerate dairy alternatives, select low oxalate options like almond milk or coconut yogurt to meet your calcium and protein needs.

- **Monitor Nut and Seed Intake:** Be cautious with nuts and seeds as they can be high in oxalates. opt for lower oxalate varieties like cashews or macadamia nuts, and consume them in moderation.

- **Supplement Wisely:** Consider consulting a healthcare provider or dietitian to determine if calcium or other nutrient supplements are necessary, especially if you have limited access to dairy or fortified products.

6.2 Low Oxalate Diet for Picky Eaters

Picky eaters may have a more limited range of food choices, making it challenging to follow a low oxalate diet. Here are some strategies to address this:

- **Identify Preferred Low Oxalate Foods:** Work with picky eaters to identify low oxalate foods they enjoy. Create meals centered around these ingredients.

- **Gradual Introduction:** Introduce new low oxalate foods slowly, one at a time. Encourage small tastes to help picky eaters become accustomed to different flavors and textures.

- **Creative Cooking:** Experiment with different cooking methods and seasonings to make low oxalate foods more appealing. Roasting, grilling, or adding herbs and spices can enhance flavors.

- **Hidden Vegetable Recipes:** Incorporate low oxalate vegetables into dishes in creative ways, such as blending them into sauces or soups to make them less noticeable.

- **Texture Matters:** Pay attention to texture preferences. Some picky eaters may prefer certain textures over others, so consider this when preparing meals.

- **Involvement in Meal Preparation:** Involve picky

eaters in meal planning and preparation. When they have a say in what's on the menu, they may be more willing to try new foods.

- **Small Changes:** Gradually make small changes to their diet by substituting high oxalate ingredients with low oxalate alternatives. Over time, this can lead to a more varied diet.

- **Be Patient:** Understand that overcoming picky eating habits takes time and patience. Avoid pressuring or forcing them to eat specific foods, as this can backfire.

- **Seek Professional Help:** If picky eating persists and affects their nutritional intake, consider consulting a registered dietitian or pediatrician for guidance and support.

Adapting to a low oxalate diet, especially as a vegetarian, vegan, or picky eater, may require some creativity and flexibility. Encourage open communication and a positive food environment to make the transition smoother and more sustainable.

CHAPTER 7

Monitoring and Adapting Your Diet

7.1 Keeping a Food Diary

Keeping a food diary is a valuable tool for monitoring and adapting your low oxalate diet. It provides insight into your dietary habits, helps you identify sources of oxalates, and allows for adjustments to better align with your health goals. Here's how to effectively maintain a food diary:

Why Keep a Food Diary:

1. **Track Oxalate Intake:** A food diary helps you keep tabs on your daily oxalate consumption, making it easier

to stay within your recommended limits.

2. **Identify Triggers:** If you have specific health concerns related to oxalates, such as kidney stones or recurring pain, a food diary can help pinpoint potential triggers by tracking symptoms alongside your diet.

3. **Assess Nutritional Balance:** You can evaluate the overall balance of your diet, ensuring you're getting the necessary nutrients while adhering to your low oxalate restrictions.

4. **Monitor Progress:** A food diary allows you to assess how well you're sticking to your low oxalate plan and whether adjustments are needed over time.

Tips for Keeping a Food Diary:

1. **Record Everything:** Write down everything you eat and drink, including portion sizes, snacks, and condiments. Be as detailed as possible.

2. **Include Preparation Methods:** Note how foods are prepared (e.g., boiled, steamed, grilled) since cooking methods can impact oxalate content.

3. **Record Symptoms:** If you have specific symptoms or reactions related to oxalates, jot them down alongside your food entries. This can help identify patterns.

4. **Use Technology:** Consider using apps or online tools designed for food tracking. These can simplify the process

and provide nutritional analysis.

5. **Set a Schedule:** Establish a routine for recording your meals. You can do this immediately after eating or at the end of the day, but consistency is key.

6. **Be Honest:** It's essential to be honest and accurate in your food diary. Include occasional indulgences or deviations from your low oxalate plan to get a complete picture.

7. **Include Beverage Intake:** Don't forget to track your fluid intake, especially water, as hydration plays a role in managing oxalates.

What to Look for in Your Food Diary:

As you maintain your food diary, pay attention to the following:

- **Oxalate Content:** Identify which foods are contributing the most oxalates to your diet. Look for patterns in high oxalate food consumption.

- **Balanced Meals:** Assess whether your meals are balanced, with a variety of low oxalate foods from different food groups.

- **Symptoms:** Note any symptoms or discomfort you experience and whether they correlate with specific foods or meals.

- **Progress:** Over time, review your food diary to see how well you're managing your low oxalate diet. Consider any necessary adjustments.

Adapting Your Diet Based on Your Food Diary:

Based on the insights from your food diary, you can make informed decisions to adapt your low oxalate diet. This might involve:

- **Identifying and Eliminating High Oxalate Culprits:** Pinpoint specific high oxalate foods or ingredients that may need to be reduced or removed from your diet.

- **Balancing Nutrient Intake:** Ensure that you're getting an adequate intake of essential nutrients, such as calcium and fiber, by adjusting your food choices.

- **Experimenting with Cooking Methods:** Modify your cooking methods to reduce oxalates in certain foods while preserving nutritional value.

- **Seeking Professional Guidance:** If you're struggling to manage your low oxalate diet or have specific medical concerns, consult with a registered dietitian or healthcare provider for personalized advice and adjustments.

Adapting your diet is an ongoing process, and your food diary serves as a valuable tool to guide you on your low oxalate journey. Regularly review and analyze your entries to make informed choices that align with your health objectives.

7.2 Tracking Your Progress

Tracking your progress on a low oxalate diet is essential for evaluating the effectiveness of your dietary choices, managing specific health conditions, and ensuring that you are meeting your health goals. Here's how to effectively track your progress:

1. Establish Clear Goals:

- Start by defining your specific goals for following a low oxalate diet. These goals could be related to reducing the risk of kidney stones, managing a medical condition, or improving overall well-being.

2. Regularly Monitor Oxalate Intake:

- Continue to maintain a detailed food diary as discussed in the previous section (7.1 Keeping a Food Diary). This will help you track your daily oxalate consumption and identify trends over time.

3. Assess Symptoms and Health Changes:

- Keep a record of any symptoms or health changes that are relevant to your low oxalate diet. This may include the frequency and severity of kidney stone episodes, digestive issues, or any other health concerns you are addressing through dietary changes.

4. Use Tracking Tools:

- Consider using technology such as mobile apps or online platforms designed for dietary tracking. These tools can provide you with insights into your nutrient intake and oxalate consumption more efficiently.

5. Periodic Reassessment:

- Periodically review your food diary, symptom journal, and any other tracking data you've collected. Look for patterns, improvements, or areas that may need adjustment.

6. Consult with Healthcare Professionals:

- If you have specific health concerns or conditions related to oxalates (e.g., recurrent kidney stones), consult with healthcare professionals, such as nephrologists or dietitians, to discuss your progress and receive guidance on any necessary changes to your dietary plan.

7. Adjust Your Diet as Needed:

- Based on your tracking and professional guidance, make informed adjustments to your low oxalate diet. This may involve further reducing high oxalate foods, experimenting with different cooking methods, or modifying portion sizes.

8. Track Nutritional Balance:

- Ensure that your low oxalate diet remains nutritionally balanced. Pay attention to your intake of essential nutrients, including calcium, vitamin D,

and fiber, to prevent
deficiencies.

9. Stay Hydrated:

- Continue to prioritize adequate hydration. Proper hydration can help reduce the risk of kidney stone formation and support overall health.

10. Celebrate Achievements:

- Acknowledge your successes and milestones. Celebrate improvements in your health, decreased symptoms, or successful adherence to your dietary plan.

11. Be Patient:

- Remember that managing a low oxalate diet is a journey that may require time and persistence. Be patient with yourself as you work toward your goals.

12. Seek Support:

- If you find it challenging to track your progress or stay motivated, consider joining support groups or seeking the assistance of a registered dietitian who specializes in low oxalate diets. Sharing experiences and receiving guidance can be highly beneficial.

Tracking your progress is a valuable tool for optimizing the benefits of a low oxalate diet and ensuring that your dietary choices align with your health objectives. Regular monitoring and adjustments will help you make informed decisions and maintain a balanced and sustainable low oxalate eating plan.

7.3 Making Adjustments as Needed

Adapting your low oxalate diet to meet your changing needs and goals is a crucial aspect of long-term success. Here's how to make adjustments as needed:

1. Regularly Review Your Progress:

- Periodically assess your progress and goals. This might be monthly, quarterly, or as determined by your healthcare provider. Review your food diary, symptom journal, and any relevant health data.

2. Consult with a Healthcare Professional:

- Maintain open communication with healthcare professionals, such as a nephrologist, urologist, or registered dietitian, who can provide guidance and monitor your health. Discuss any changes in your condition or dietary challenges.

3. Modify Your Oxalate Intake:

- Based on your progress and professional advice, adjust your oxalate intake as necessary. This might involve increasing or decreasing the amount of high oxalate foods in your diet.

4. Experiment with Cooking Methods:

- Explore different cooking methods to reduce oxalates in high oxalate foods while preserving their nutritional value. For instance, try boiling or blanching vegetables instead of eating them raw.

5. Try Oxalate Binders (Under Medical Supervision):

- If you have a medical condition that requires strict oxalate control, discuss the possibility of using oxalate binders with your healthcare provider. These medications can help reduce oxalate absorption in the intestines.

6. Monitor Nutritional Balance:

- Ensure that your low oxalate diet continues to provide essential nutrients. Pay attention to your intake of calcium, vitamin D, and other vital nutrients to prevent deficiencies.

7. Be Mindful of Food Combinations:

- Consider how different foods interact in your diet. Some combinations can enhance or inhibit oxalate absorption. For instance, consuming calcium-rich foods alongside high oxalate foods may help reduce oxalate absorption.

8. Adapt to Changing Dietary Preferences:

- If your dietary preferences change over time, adjust your low oxalate diet accordingly. For example, if you transition from vegetarianism to a non-vegetarian diet, your food choices will shift.

9. Address New Health Concerns:

- If you develop new health concerns or conditions, consult with healthcare professionals to incorporate them into your dietary plan. Certain conditions may necessitate further dietary restrictions or adjustments.

10. Stay Hydrated: - Maintain proper hydration to support overall kidney health. Drinking an adequate amount of water can help dilute oxalates and reduce the risk of kidney stone formation.

11. Evaluate Medication Interactions: - If you are taking medications that may interact with oxalates or affect your dietary needs, discuss this with your healthcare provider. They can help you make informed adjustments.

12. Be Patient and Flexible: - Understand that dietary adjustments are an ongoing process. Be patient and adaptable as you fine-tune your low oxalate diet to meet your changing needs and health circumstances.

13. Seek Support: - If you find it challenging to make adjustments or need guidance, consider seeking support from a registered dietitian with expertise in low oxalate diets. They can provide personalized advice and meal planning assistance.

Making adjustments to your low oxalate diet is a dynamic process. Regular monitoring, consultation with healthcare professionals, and a willingness to adapt will help you

maintain a balanced and effective
dietary plan that aligns with your
health goals and evolving needs.

CHAPTER 8

Potential Benefits and Considerations

8.1 Health Benefits of a Low Oxalate Diet

A low oxalate diet may offer several health benefits, especially for individuals with specific medical conditions or concerns related to oxalates. Here are some potential health benefits of following a low oxalate diet:

1. Kidney Stone Prevention:

- Reduced oxalate intake can decrease the risk of calcium oxalate kidney stone formation, one of the most common types of kidney stones. By limiting the dietary source of oxalates, individuals prone to kidney stones may experience a lower incidence of stone recurrence.

2. Management of Hyperoxaluria:

- For individuals with primary or secondary hyperoxaluria, a low oxalate diet can help manage excessive oxalate levels in the body, potentially reducing the risk of kidney damage and complications associated with oxalate accumulation.

3. Symptom Relief in Certain Conditions:

- Some individuals with conditions like interstitial cystitis or vulvodynia may experience symptom relief by reducing dietary oxalates.

Lower oxalate intake may help alleviate pain and discomfort in these conditions.

4. Improved Digestive Health:

- For individuals with gastrointestinal conditions that may be exacerbated by high oxalate intake, such as irritable bowel syndrome (IBS) or inflammatory bowel disease (IBD), a low oxalate diet can reduce symptoms like abdominal pain and diarrhea.

5. Enhanced Nutritional Balance:

- A well-planned low oxalate diet can encourage individuals to focus on nutrient-dense foods, such as fruits, vegetables, lean proteins, and whole grains. This can promote overall nutritional balance and health.

6. Tailored Dietary Management:

- A low oxalate diet can be tailored to the specific needs and tolerances of individuals. This flexibility allows for dietary customization to address individual health concerns.

7. Potential Reduction in Oxalate-Related Symptoms:

- Some individuals may experience symptoms related to oxalate sensitivity, such as joint pain, skin rashes, or recurring urinary tract infections. Reducing dietary oxalates may alleviate these symptoms.

8. Personalized Nutritional Support:

- A low oxalate diet can be an essential part of personalized nutritional support for individuals with certain medical conditions. Healthcare providers and dietitians can guide individuals in optimizing their dietary choices.

while a low oxalate diet can offer health benefits for some individuals, it may not be suitable or necessary for everyone. The decision to follow a low oxalate diet should be made in consultation with a healthcare provider or registered dietitian, who can provide personalized guidance based on individual health concerns, dietary preferences, and nutritional needs. Additionally, it's important to ensure that any dietary restrictions do not lead to nutrient deficiencies or other adverse effects on overall health.

8.2 Potential Risks and Considerations

While a low oxalate diet can offer benefits for certain individuals, it's essential to be aware of potential risks and considerations associated with this dietary approach:

1. Nutritional Imbalance:

- Restricting high oxalate foods may lead to a reduced intake of essential nutrients, such as dietary fiber, vitamins, and minerals, including calcium. This can potentially increase the risk of nutritional deficiencies if the diet is not carefully planned.

2. Impact on Gut Health:

- Some low oxalate diets may inadvertently reduce the consumption of high-fiber foods, which are essential for gut health. This can affect digestion and overall gastrointestinal well-being.

3. Difficulty Achieving Adequate Calcium Intake:

- Limiting dairy products (which are high in calcium) due to their oxalate content can make it challenging to meet daily calcium requirements. Calcium is essential for bone health, and inadequate intake can lead to osteoporosis or other bone-related issues.

4. Limited Food Choices:

- A low oxalate diet can be restrictive, potentially leading to monotony and boredom with food choices. This may make it challenging to maintain the diet long-term.

5. Variability in Oxalate Content:

- Oxalate content can vary among foods and even within the same type of food, depending on factors like variety, ripeness, and processing. This variability can make it difficult to accurately estimate oxalate intake.

6. Potential for Ineffective Management:

- For some individuals, a low oxalate diet may not effectively prevent kidney stones or alleviate related symptoms.

Other underlying factors, such as hydration, urinary pH, and medication, also play a significant role in stone formation.

7. Lack of Evidence for Some Conditions:

- While a low oxalate diet is well-established for managing kidney stones and certain medical conditions, its effectiveness for addressing other oxalate-related symptoms is less clear. Scientific evidence may be limited in some cases.

8. Social and Lifestyle Impacts:

- Adhering to a strict low oxalate diet can affect social and lifestyle aspects, including dining out, family gatherings, and cultural traditions. These

impacts should be considered
when making dietary choices.

9. Individual Variation:

- Oxalate tolerance varies among
  individuals. Some people may
  tolerate higher oxalate intake
  without adverse effects, while
  others may be more sensitive to
  oxalates.

8.3 Consulting with a Healthcare Professional

Before starting or significantly
modifying your diet, especially a low
oxalate diet, it's crucial to consult with
a healthcare professional, such as a
registered dietitian or a specialist in
nephrology or urology. Here's why
consulting with a healthcare
professional is important:

1. Personalized Guidance:

- Healthcare professionals can provide personalized dietary guidance based on your specific health concerns, medical history, and nutritional needs.

2. Comprehensive Evaluation:

- They can perform a comprehensive evaluation to determine whether a low oxalate diet is appropriate for your individual situation or if other treatments or dietary modifications are necessary.

3. Nutritional Balance:

- Healthcare professionals can help you create a balanced low oxalate diet that ensures you receive essential nutrients and

minimizes the risk of
nutritional deficiencies.

4. Monitoring and Assessment:

- They can monitor your progress
  and assess the effectiveness of
  the diet in managing your
  health condition, making
  necessary adjustments as
  needed.

5. Addressing Concerns:

- If you have concerns or
  questions about the low oxalate
  diet, healthcare professionals
  can address them, provide
  evidence-based information,
  and clarify misconceptions.

6. Avoiding Unnecessary Restrictions:

- Consulting with a healthcare
  professional can help you avoid

unnecessary dietary restrictions
and ensure that dietary changes
align with your health goals
and needs.

7. Long-Term Success:

- Healthcare professionals can
  assist in creating a sustainable
  dietary plan that promotes long-
  term success and minimizes the
  potential risks associated with a
  low oxalate diet.

Healthcare professionals can provide
valuable guidance and support to help
you make informed decisions about
your diet and overall health. Their
expertise is essential in ensuring that
dietary changes are both effective and
safe.